?
what's your excuse
for not eating
healthily

what's your excuse ...

FOR NOT

EATING HEALTHILY

Overcome your excuses and eat well to look good and feel great

joanne henson

"Very useful, very practical and makes a lot of sense! There are some great tips in here and even if you just implemented a bit of Joanne's advice it would make a real difference"

"I will certainly be using this as a reference book and keeping it handy at all times. I enjoyed it immensely and was very excited that someone was talking my language. I would highly recommend it if you struggle to eat well for a sustained period. I guarantee you will be nodding in agreement whilst turning the pages"

"A concise answer for a wide range of popular excuses for eating junk and avoiding your five-a-day …. ideal for those moments when you hear yourself making a crappy excuse and need your butt kicked to get you back on track!"

"It's like you're having a conversation with one of those people who doesn't take any of your shit. Reading these books is like someone holding up a big mirror to your whining, excuse-making, sorry self. Joanne has an answer for every excuse, so you're left with '… er… ok. I'll join the gym and buy some *apples'. And then… the books sit there and taunt you…There's nothing in these books that's ground breaking but that's the beauty of them. They tell you everything you already knew, in language you can understand. They're like that voice in your head that's usually drowned out by your expert excuse-maker voice"*

singlemotherahoy.com

Also in the series

What's Your Excuse for not....

Getting Fit?
Living a Life You Love?

What's Your Excuse for not Eating Healthily?

Second edition
Published by WYE Publishing 2015
www.wyepublishing.com

First published in 2014 by Completely Novel

ISBN 978-0-9933388-2-3

Cover and text design by Annette Peppis & Associates

Printed in UK by Marston Book Services Ltd, Oxfordshire

'What's Your Excuse.....?' is a UK Registered Trade Mark (Registration No: 3018995)

www.whatsyourexcuse.co.uk
Follow What's Your Excuse.....? on Twitter - @whats_yr_excuse

www.joannehenson.co.uk
Follow Joanne on Twitter - @joannemh

Contents

Introduction

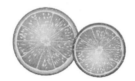

How to use this book

Welcome to *What's Your Excuse for not Eating Healthily?*

This book is not yet another diet book. I am not going to set out eating plans, nor tell you what to eat and what not to eat. But I will help you improve your eating habits.

If you've ever embarked on a diet, or simply tried to improve how you eat, you'll know that it's not always easy. You'll experience periods of high motivation, but these will be interspersed with times when the temptation to eat a treat is just too great, or when you just don't seem to be making the right food choices.

As a health and wellness coach I have helped many clients to improve their diet and their wellbeing, and one of the key things I do with them is to examine the excuses they use, so that I can work with them to overcome their own personal obstacles and sticking points.

I have heard the same set of excuses from my clients over and over again. I used to use some of these excuses myself. What I've compiled here is a collection of every excuse I have ever heard, with suggestions on how to overcome them. When you've read my ideas, they might spark some further ones of your own – it's all about creative thinking and looking at problems from new angles.

You may want to read this book from cover to cover to absorb its positive messages and kick-start a move towards a better way of eating. It will certainly give you that motivation - read the next chapter to remind yourself of the benefits of healthy eating to set the scene.

But this book is also designed as a handy reference guide and quick fix for those moments when you find yourself at risk of abandoning your resolve to eat well, or reaching for a sugary snack out of habit, boredom or any other reason. When you feel an excuse coming on, look it up and read the tips on how to tackle what's going on in your head. Then set the excuse to one side and continue your journey towards a healthier, happier you, with a more positive relationship with food.

And if you find yourself coming up with innovative and creative excuses which do not appear in this book, I would love to hear from you – I will incorporate them into the next edition!

Finally, if you are struggling to stick with an exercise regime too, take a look at my book *"What's Your Excuse for not Getting Fit?"*

The benefits of eating healthily

Before you move on to the excuses, it's worth reminding yourself of your reasons for wanting to eat well in the first place.

Research shows over and over again that when you have a goal, the more you remind yourself of its benefits, and the more you visualise how it will feel when you get there, the more inspired you will be to continue to work towards it.

So find a notepad and take a few minutes to jot down the reasons why you want to improve the way you eat. This will be your own personal Benefits List.

If you're stuck, here are some ideas:

- I will have more energy
- I will feel and look better in my clothes
- I won't be embarrassed to get naked in front of my partner
- My health problems will improve and I may be able to reduce my medication

- I will feel more positive
- I might live longer
- I won't have to shop in plus size stores
- My skin will glow
- I will have a better relationship with food
- I'll receive compliments
- I'll know that I am taking care of myself
- I may lose weight
- I'll see better results in the gym
- I'll prove all those people wrong who said I couldn't do it
- I'll inspire those around me to improve their health too
- I will no longer consider myself incapable of eating well
- I'll have abs instead of a belly
- I will like myself
- I'll know that I have overcome my excuses!

From now on, whenever you find yourself about to use an excuse to make a poor food choice, take a look at your Benefits List to remind you of your ultimate goal and of how you will feel if you set that excuse to one side and move on.

The consequences of eating unhealthily

The previous chapter was intended to emphasise how life can be so much better if you're operating from a healthy foundation.

If you need further encouragement here are some of the things you might experience if you have an unhealthy diet:

- You may have no energy or experience energy slumps
- You may have cravings for sugary snacks
- You'll be more likely to develop diseases such as diabetes and heart disease
- You might not like what you see when you look in the mirror
- You could feel like you have no willpower
- Your hair, skin and nails might look dull
- Your clothes could feel tight and uncomfortable
- You could feel guilty
- You might have to shop in plus-size shops
- People might keep telling you how tired you look
- You're more likely to have cellulite
- You might not age well

- You'll be more susceptible to picking up colds and other viruses

Feel free to add more of your own!

A note about the word "diet"

The word "diet" started out simply as a way to describe what we eat – the Oxford English Dictionary defines it as "the kinds of food that a person, animal or community habitually eats".

However common parlance generally has the word used in the context of a weight loss regime.

Throughout this book I will be using the word in its original sense. Where I use it to refer to a weight loss regime I will express it as a Diet.

A note about the definition of healthy eating

With so much research being undertaken into foods and their effects on our bodies, there will always be conflicting opinion and advice on what is healthy and what isn't.

The purpose of this book is not to examine current theories on nutrition, nor is it to promote a particular way of eating, but for the record, these are what I believe to be the key elements of healthy eating:

- Low sugar
- High proportion of fresh foods
- Sufficient healthy fat
- Sufficient protein
- Sufficient fibre
- Minimal artificial additives and sweeteners
- Minimal amount of processed foods

The other key element of healthy eating is to eat the right amount of food. This means not too much, but just as importantly not too little. Getting very skinny is not healthy.

Many of my coaching clients have a background of yoyo dieting, and come to me with the belief that healthy eating is as much about reducing the quantity of their food as it is about improving the quality. In fact, unless binge eating is an issue for you, if you improve the quality of your diet you might find that you won't need to worry about reducing the quantity, even if you have weight to lose.

The Excuses

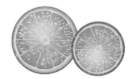

Mind

I've got no willpower

You only need willpower when you're being tempted. If you're not being tempted and there's no possibility of you reaching for unhealthy food or eating too much food, then you don't need willpower.

So, in environments which you can control, like your own home and possibly your office, try to remove temptation. If you don't want to find yourself eating crisps out of boredom in front of the TV in the evening, don't have crisps in the house. If you don't want to find yourself eating a whole packet of chocolate biscuits in one sitting, buy individually wrapped ones, one at a time[1]. Then it doesn't matter if you have no willpower – you won't need it, there'll be nothing to tempt you anyway.

But what if you live with a partner and he/she likes to have treats in the house? You'll say you can't ban

---

1   I acknowledge that buying single portions of food is more expensive than buying a family size pack, or getting three for the price of two, but if you're not struggling for cash then view the extra spend as an investment in your health. And remember that buying a family sized pack of something to save money but then eating it all in one sitting isn't an economy anyway!

them from having treats around if they aren't joining you in your new way of eating. How about identifying some foods which are treats for them but which you don't enjoy? I used to be tempted by the biscuits which my partner liked to have around the house, until I realised that there were others he liked equally which I don't like. So I got him to buy a different brand, which didn't tempt me at all - problem solved.

And if you have a family? I appreciate that kids can be very specific about what they do and don't like, but once again are there things that they like to eat which you don't, and which would therefore be "safe" to have around the house? And do they really need the treats every week? I'm not about to start preaching about how kids should be eating healthily but if your house is full of unhealthy snacks for your family could you at least reduce the quantity?

So that's one way to get around a lack of willpower – minimise the need for it. And get creative about that. If you are tempted by the bread basket when you're eating out, ask your friends to put it at the other end of the table, out of your reach. And if your friends don't want the temptation either, ask the server to take it away. If you know you'll be tempted by the cakes on display when you go into a coffee shop, ask whoever you're with to go to the counter, and go straight to the table, with your back to the counter if that's what it takes. What's your own personal temptation and what can you do to remove it from view or put it further out of reach?

There are however going to be times and places when you can't control what's around you, when you will need to find the willpower to restrain yourself and make healthy choices. In these cases, it helps to *focus, focus, focus* - you will be most successful when you have your end goal fixed firmly in your mind. Remind yourself why you want to

> What's your own personal temptation and what can you do to remove it from view or put it further out of reach?

avoid sugary snacks, too much alcohol, processed foods, or whatever temptation you're facing at the time. *You want that end result so much that you're willing to put the effort in to get it.* If you made a Benefits List as I suggested at the beginning of this book, take a look at it. There's a saying, "Begin with the end in mind" but I think it's more about *progressing* with the end in mind. *Remind yourself all the time why you are doing this.*

Also, try to surround yourself with supportive and positive people. If your friends are constantly trying to tempt you to eat what they know you don't want to eat, then are they really the people you need around you? Ask for their support and if they are good friends they should be willing to give it.

Finally, when you've given in to a sugary snack and you're beating yourself up because you think your willpower has failed you, ask yourself what you ate last. Was it high sugar? All too often my clients beat themselves up for giving in to temptation when in fact they've been battling a blood sugar low which has made it pretty much impossible to resist more sugar. If you have a high carbohydrate snack or meal, don't be surprised if shortly afterwards your energy levels slump and your mind turns to food – the food you chose gave you a blood sugar spike followed by a low, which then causes cravings which you translate as a lack of willpower. Just realising this has helped many of my clients stop feeling guilty about their sugar cravings, and once they've been able to stop beating themselves up they've been able to think more clearly about their food choices.

Surround yourself with supportive and positive people.

If you think blood sugar fluctuations might be your problem, try protein-based breakfasts. This will give you a stable start to your day, which may be all it takes to break the cycle of craving and giving in to unhealthy snacks.

I'm too stressed to think about healthy food

One of the people I interviewed for this book has a high pressure, stressful job, followed by an all-too-often stressful commute. She told me that when she gets home from work she is too mentally worn out to make decisions about what to cook, even though her fridge is full of fruit and vegetables. So she makes herself a fish finger sandwich and the fruit and vegetables get thrown away at the end of the week.

I am sympathetic to anyone who has to deal with stress – it's draining, and leaves people with little mental energy to do exactly the thing they should be doing, which is taking care of themselves. So while I am sympathetic (and I lived through a very stressful couple of years during which I didn't practice what I preach) I would urge you to find ways of eating healthily to counteract the corrosive effects of stress.

So you're standing in your kitchen, exhausted by the day's work and too tired to think about creating a healthy meal. What can you do? Well, firstly, just because you don't feel like creating a healthy home cooked meal you don't automatically have to reach for the least healthy food in the house. Some vegetable soup or a slice of wholemeal toast with peanut butter followed by a piece of fruit would be better than, say, a packet of biscuits or a pizza delivery and would take only a couple of minutes to prepare.

If this is a common scenario for you, start planning in advance for these moments. Do you own a freezer and a microwave? Spend some time at the weekend cooking up some healthy meals which you can freeze and then microwave when you need them. If you prepare one dish a week, and freeze a few portions, over the weeks you'll build up a variety of different things to choose from.

And consider not having unhealthy options in the house – no fish fingers in the freezer, no possibility of fish finger sandwiches! See "I've got no willpower" for more on this.

> Be prepared and have some healthy snacks in your bag or desk.

If your problem is stress during the day (rather than when you get home), again remember that just because you don't ever take a lunch break or have the time to go out and buy or prepare a nutritious lunch it doesn't mean that your only option has to be chocolate and crisps from a vending machine. Be prepared and have some healthy snacks in your bag or desk – buy them at the weekend, take them in on a Monday, job done for the week. Snacking on the go might not be perfect, but it's better than not eating at all, or resorting to eating rubbish.

I get cravings

When do you get these cravings? Is it at a particular time of day? The most common craving seems to be the mid-afternoon energy slump – you had your lunch two hours earlier and now you're craving chocolate. Well guess what? That craving could well be a result of what you ate for lunch. Did you have a jacket potato, soup with bread, or a sandwich or baguette? If your lunch comprised more carbohydrate than fat or protein it will have caused your blood sugar level to rise and then fall. And now it's fallen, your body is craving more food to fix that.

Nick Owen, a nutritional therapist, says, "Clients who complain of cravings are usually clients who don't eat breakfast, or who don't eat regularly". That is, clients with fluctuating blood sugar.

So your cravings are very likely to be caused by your general eating patterns, rather than an inbuilt desire for chocolate, fries, pizza or whatever else it is you hanker after. And it *is* usually high-calorie, high-sugar food which people crave – I very rarely hear people say they suffer from cravings for vegetables or a grilled chicken breast.

Many people think the only fix for cravings is simply to resist. Except they usually aren't able to, or they make themselves miserable trying, because the chemicals and hormones in their bodies are working against them. The fix is a long-term one - improve your overall eating patterns, to rid yourself of the physical craving so there'll be nothing to resist, and no more feeling guilty about giving in as there'll be nothing to give in to.

So far, so good. But when I ask my clients to explain to me what's going on for them when a craving starts, there's often something else going on – habit. Let's say you've improved the way you eat at lunchtime, and mid-afternoon your body is no longer crying out for an energy hit, because your blood sugar levels are more stable. But if over the last couple of years you've been getting up from your desk at 3pm, stretching your legs, making a cup of tea, having a chat to a colleague in the kitchen and then settling back down at your desk with your tea and a handful of biscuits, those biscuits which you first started eating to fix your low energy levels have now become part of a habit, or ritual.

> A good way of breaking a bad habit is to replace it with a different, better one.

A good way of breaking a bad habit is to replace it with a different, better one. One of my coaching clients said that she always craved biscuits whenever she made a cup of tea. Her solution? To make a coffee instead, as she doesn't like eating biscuits with coffee.

Another way to break a habit is to change the pattern of events which lead up to it. A friend of mine used to walk from the office to the bus stop at the end of her working day, and call in to the newsagents for a bar of chocolate on her way. To break this habit she chose to walk the other way, to a different bus stop, which was not much further, but importantly didn't involve passing a newsagent.

What could you change to break an unhealthy habit?

See also "I just can't resist...." and "I always have a treat mid-afternoon/I always have a fry-up on a Sunday".

I don't have the motivation

Are you saying that you've never had the motivation in the past? Or that you don't have it now?

Let's take a look at the past first. *Your past does not equal your future,* but it may do, if you don't work out what tripped you up last time and if you don't make some changes. Just because you've failed in an attempt to improve your diet before does not mean that you'll fail again. But you are more likely to fail if you don't change something this time around – *if you always do what you've always done you'll always get what you always got.*

So have a think about what didn't work for you last time. Not what *you* did wrong, but what didn't work *for you* – there is a big difference. Were you on a Diet which didn't suit your lifestyle, or which was too restrictive? Then of course you won't have been motivated. Find a way of eating which suits you, and once you do you won't need motivation as it won't feel difficult. Keep reading to learn lots more about how to make healthy eating work for you.

If you're saying that you just don't have the motivation right now, *focus, focus, focus* – keep your eye on the prize, focus on the rewards. For instance, which you do want more, a second piece of cake or to fit into that new dress for your birthday party? If you completed a Benefits List as I suggested at the start of this book take a look at it. There are your rewards. There is your motivation. Carry it with you and look at it, often.

See also "I've got no willpower".

I'm having a really bad time at the moment

If it's just one bad day, then see the next excuse, "I'm having a bad day".

If you're going through a difficult time in your life

healthy eating might not be your top priority, and that's understandable. But that doesn't mean that you have to go to the other extreme and abandon all attempts to eat well. Try to stick with at least some healthy habits – drink enough water, eat regularly, get some fresh fruit and vegetables, whatever you can manage.

The one thing you do still have control over is what you eat.

If you're feeling out of control at work, or in your relationships, or in any other area of your life consider this: the one thing you do still have control over is what you eat, and although you might not have masses of energy to devote to buying and preparing nutritious food, try to see healthy eating as something you can do for yourself which no one else can take away from you. If you can do this it will help to combat the effects of those things you can't control. You will be far more physically resilient to stress if you're feeling well-nourished, and you'll be far more mentally resilient if you aren't also beating yourself up over succumbing to cakes and biscuits.

Take care of yourself.

I've had a bad day

One bad day is no big deal and if you want to go home, put on your pyjamas and pour yourself a glass of wine you'll do yourself no long term damage.

But if you're saying this a lot see "I'm having a really bad time at the moment" above.

Or are you getting home after a day's work and feeling like you deserve a treat, as a reward for your hard work? See "I deserved a treat".

Food

Healthy food is boring

When clients tell me that they find healthy food boring, I ask them to give me some examples. These are some of the more common answers I get:

- Cottage cheese (particularly the low fat version)
- Yoghurt (once again, usually a low fat version)
- Rice cakes
- Low calorie cereals
- Lettuce
- Low calorie/low fat ready meals
- Calorie counted sandwiches
- Skimmed milk
- Lower fat or baked crisps

They all sound pretty boring to me too, and I don't eat them.

In fact none of those items are particularly healthy. They are just low calorie and/or low fat, which is a very different thing. Low calorie or low fat foods are more processed than the normal versions and have less flavour, although manufacturers usually try to compensate for the lack of flavour by adding additional sugar, artificial flavourings and sometimes salt, none of which is going to do you any good.

So if you find a food boring, don't eat it. Healthy food can be tasty and satisfying, and if you shop around and try new foods, you'll find a massive variety of interesting flavours and textures to enjoy.

I'm a chocoholic

You love chocolate and the implication here is that you are simply unable to resist it because it's so addictive.

Well, chocolate does contain a number of mood enhancing substances (phenylethylamine, theobromine, anandamide, tryptophan), and they've all been the subject of many studies to ascertain whether they cause chocolate to be an addictive substance. The general consensus however is that these chemicals are present in such small quantities that they have no real effect. In fact, these chemicals are found in much higher concentrations in less appealing foods, none of which are claimed to be addictive.

I've also heard claims that people feel addicted to chocolate because they are deficient in magnesium, and that they are naturally drawn to chocolate because it contains magnesium. In fact many other foods such as green leafy vegetables contain much higher levels but no one ever claims to be addicted to spinach.

But chocolate is not off the hook yet, because it does contain something very addictive, in significant quantities – sugar. And it's likely that your cravings for chocolate are mainly related to this. If you find yourself having one bar of chocolate only to want another one shortly afterwards, it's the sugar that's getting to you. Immediately after one sugary snack your blood sugar will rise rapidly and then fall. As it falls, you will find yourself craving another sugar hit, and if you have another one the blood sugar high and low will happen again, and so the cycle will continue. It will feel like an addiction.

If this strikes a chord with you, try including some protein in each of your meals to alleviate these extreme blood sugar fluctuations. A meal which includes sufficient protein won't cause a blood sugar spike, so there won't be a rapid fall either, nor any sudden subsequent sugar cravings.

I have one more observation on this "addiction": generally, when people declare themselves to be chocoholics, they do so with a smile, and sometimes with thinly veiled pride. So if you're one of those people, ask yourself this - are you using this term simply to give yourself permission to indulge in chocolate more often than you know you should? Try to stop using the term for a while, and see how it feels to say, "I eat lots of chocolate" instead. Bet that doesn't feel quite so good.

I need to prepare food which the kids will eat

It takes a while for kids to acquire the taste for something. Just because they say they don't like it the first time doesn't mean they won't like it a second time if it is served differently.

My sister used to hate vegetables when she was young. Our Mum would put our meals in front of us and immediately my sister would ask if she could leave her vegetables. Our Mum's response was always, "If you have to leave something, you can leave some of the mashed potato" (there was always mashed potato)[2]. My sister thought she was clever though. She hated cauliflower, so when Mum's back was turned she would disguise it in her mashed potato, which she left on her plate. It didn't fool Mum for long, and soon she was back to being encouraged to eat her vegetables at every meal. And by being (firmly) encouraged to eat our

---

2   Good advice from Mum there – eat the nutritious vegetables in preference to the white carbs

vegetables, by the time we were teenagers my sister and I happily ate all sorts of vegetables. In fact my sister is now vegetarian, eats about 10 portions of vegetables every day, and grows them on her own allotment. She's never managed to successfully grow cauliflowers though.

Should your children really dictate what you eat?

I'm telling you this because I see many parents allowing their children to pick and choose what they eat, and allowing them to say no to healthy food. And if they aren't eating healthy food then they are eating processed food, which you could well end up eating with them. And should your children really dictate what you eat?

If your kids don't like healthy foods in one form, get creative. They might not like steamed vegetables, but they might like vegetable soup. They might not like tomatoes but they might eat homemade tomato sauce. There are whole recipe books dedicated to making healthy food appealing to children – try "The Top 100 Recipes for Happy Kids: Keep Your Child Alert, Focused and Active" by Charlotte Watts, or Anita Bean's "Healthy Eating for Kids". Your kids should be eating as healthily as you.

And if all else fails you could always disguise their vegetables in the mashed potato.

I just can't resist....

We all have our food nemesis. I just can't resist peanut butter. Now I know as favourite foods go that's not so bad, but it is when it's eaten in large quantities direct from the jar with a spoon, when I am not even hungry and in between meals. However you only need to resist something if it's there to be resisted. So I don't always have peanut butter in the house. And when I do, I buy the smallest jar I can, and really try to savour it. I make it an occasional treat rather than a constant temptation.

Don't attempt to give up your favourite food totally. We should all have a treat from time to time. But try to make it just that – a *treat,* not something you indulge in all the time so that it's tied up with feelings of guilt. If you can't resist crisps, don't have them in the house. Or if you have a family and you have to have them in the house because your partner or kids want to eat them, can you ask them to choose flavours or brands you don't like?

And then when you do have your occasional treat, make it an event, savour it and *don't feel guilty.*

See also "I've got no willpower".

I don't like leaving leftovers

Like most people, I was brought up to clear my plate (with the occasional exception of mashed potato – see "I need to prepare food which the kids will eat"). I was taught that it was wasteful and ungrateful to leave food. And after years of being programmed in that way, many adults find that they go into plate-clearing auto-pilot mode at mealtimes, without ever stopping to consider whether they have actually had enough. Coupled with a general trend towards bigger portions, at home and when eating out, our plate-clearing habits are causing us to regularly eat more than we need.

Our behaviour was shaped when we were children, when our parents were buying preparing, cooking and serving the food. But we are now adults, who can choose to buy, prepare, cook, serve and eat as much or as little food as we like, so we have every opportunity to avoid those leftovers situations.

There are two main options to tackle an issue with leftovers – you can put less on your plate in the first place, or you can give yourself permission to throw away any excess.

To put less on your plate, just cook less. Or, taking a step further back, *buy* less at the supermarket. That really would be eliminating waste. And since we're all now surrounded by mini-supermarkets which open long hours seven days a week there's no need to stock-pile food in the house. Buy less, cook less, eat less. If that means you have to shop a little more often, great, you'll be eating fresher food too.

Your second option is to give yourself permission to leave excess food on your plate, and to throw it away. Does that sound difficult? Well here's a thought for you - eating food which you don't need or want is *just as wasteful* as throwing it away – either way, it's wasted, and isn't going to good use.

Our plate-clearing habits are causing us to regularly eat more than we need.

If you're in a restaurant and you're served an enormous plate of food, you're doing no one any favours by forcing yourself to finish it - either way, the excess wouldn't be finding its way onto the plate of a starving orphan, it's going in the restaurant's bin (although I suppose there's a chance an urban fox might benefit from it).

Finally, ask yourself this: when you make the statement "I can't leave leftovers" are you actually just giving yourself permission to eat more than you know you need? Are you making a virtue out of eating too much? Try to refrain from saying it, to yourself and to others, so that it doesn't become a self-fulfilling prophecy.

I eat the kid's leftovers

If your kids are eating healthily then I'm not sure it's so bad to finish up the last vegetable or last piece of fruit on their plate as you clear the table.

But if it's chips, chicken nuggets or pizza slices you're polishing off, how can you reduce the opportunity to pick up food from their plates? How about getting the kids to clear away their own plates, and put whatever is left in the bin before you get a chance to eat it?

And do you really like this food that you're eating as a means of clearing it away, turning your body into a dustbin? Save yourself for something you actually enjoy.

I'm tired and need a sugar hit

Lack of sleep affects your body's hormone balance so that your appetite increases, particularly for high calorie foods. It causes a reduction in leptin (the hormone involved in telling you when you are full) and an elevation in ghrelin (the hormone involved in telling you you're hungry), so you're not getting the right messages from your body about food. Lack of sleep also raises cortisol levels, which encourages your body to store fat, and decreases levels of serotonin, which can lead to depression and (you guessed it) overeating. So if you're tired you really will be craving a sugar hit, and you'll be struggling to make wise food choices because your hormones are so out of kilter.

Lack of sleep raises cortisol levels, which encourages your body to store fat.

There's really only one solution to this, which is to increase the amount of quality sleep you get.

If you are short on sleep because you regularly stay up late just because you can, or because you love to party, then if you're serious about improving your diet and all the benefits that will bring it's time to make more of a priority of sleep. Plan a couple of early nights each week, put them in your diary, and enjoy feeling refreshed the next day.

If you go to bed at a reasonable time but struggle to get to sleep, or wake up throughout the night, try making some changes to your routine or environment. Have your last cup of coffee of the day earlier, don't eat a big meal late in the evening, don't have a TV in your bedroom, don't take a laptop to bed or pick up work emails in bed, don't do a challenging workout too late in the evening, try a black-out blind, create a calm environment in your bedroom, establish a regular sleep pattern, have a warm bath before bed. You may need to try a few different things before you find something which works for you, but there are hundreds of self-help books available on this subject.

The key thing is not to underestimate the importance of sleep. If you're well rested, you are much less likely to reach for high calorie, processed, sugary foods.

I'm on my own and it's not worth cooking for one

When you bought this book, whose health were you hoping to improve? I'm guessing it's your own. So if you're faced with preparing food just for yourself, tell me, why wouldn't it be worth preparing something nutritious?

Some of my clients who live on their own tell me that they are put off by recipes which serve 4, but it's always possible to reduce quantities to make a single portion, or to make four portions and freeze the rest for days when you really don't feel like cooking.

And if you really don't feel like preparing a meal, then fine, but that isn't a licence to eat junk – you can have a no-cook snack which is still healthy.

Eating on your own is actually a fantastic opportunity to eat what you love and what will make you feel good, all of the time. Compared to parents, who have to conjure up dishes which they, their partner and their children like, it's a privilege to be able to eat on your own, to have the freedom to make selfish choices and to enjoy exactly what you want to eat on any given day. Make the most of it!

I always have a treat mid-afternoon/I always have a fry-up on a Sunday

Healthy eating does not have to be 100% perfect eating. So if, once a week, you have a treat which you really look forward to, and you're eating well at all other times, enjoy!

But some people have numerous regular unhealthy habits:

"I always like a drink after work on a Friday"
"We always do a family fry-up on Saturday morning"
"I always have a biscuit with my cup of tea at three o'clock"
"I always buy a can of Coke on my way into work in the morning"
"I always have a grande latte with cream on top when my colleagues do a coffee run"

"I always treat myself to a bar of chocolate when I go to the petrol station"
"We always share a pizza and garlic bread in front of the TV on a Saturday night"

All of these statements have one thing in common – "always". But they don't have to be always. They could be occasional or fortnightly or monthly.

If you're guilty of having multiple unhealthy habits or rituals you will need to consider how you can reduce the damage done, or reduce the frequency. So could the latte, can of coke or biscuits be a Friday treat rather than a daily one, could the Friday night trip to the pub be for one drink not two (or three or four), could the shared pizza be a shared meal prepared from fresh ingredients (you can still share it on the sofa in front of the TV in your onesies)? Could the latte be a small one, without cream? Could the fry-up be a healthier version?

If you want to feel and look fantastic then you do need to eat well *most* of the time. So take a look at your habits and make a deal with yourself – what are the treats you most want to keep in your life, and in order to do that, what are you willing to give up? And then when you've decided on the habits you're happy to ditch, what can you do to divert yourself from the chain of events that leads up them, or what can you do instead?

I couldn't leave the packet half-finished

I am assuming it was a packet of something high in sugar or salt? Those foods are formulated to be delicious and moreish so you do keep buying more. Sugar in particular can trigger your hormones to want more even before it's been absorbed into your bloodstream. So this is not just about a lack of willpower or a weakness on your part, it's about how your body's chemicals are reacting to the first biscuit, crisp, chocolate or sweet you put in your mouth. Based on this, what can you do to avoid finding yourself at the mercy of a whole packet again? Can you buy single portions, or share the packet, or leave half of the packet in the office or at home?

See also "I've got no willpower".

If you couldn't leave the food half-finished because you don't like leaving leftovers, well, if you put food away for tomorrow then it's not leftover or wasted, it's *saved* for later. But see "I don't like leaving leftovers" earlier in this book for more on this.

Weather

It's cold so I need comfort food

"Comfort food" generally seems to mean something hot, in a bowl, eaten with just a spoon or a fork. But that often translates into high-carbohydrate, high calorie dishes with little nutritional value such as pasta, puddings and pies.

When it's cold, dark and wet outside of course it's great to get cosy at home with a warm meal but there are lots of nutritious comforting options - chunky soups, stews, casseroles, roast winter vegetables, spiced winter fruits. Food doesn't have to be unhealthy to provide comfort and warmth.

Where's the comfort in emerging from your winter woollies in Spring feeling sluggish and no longer fitting into your jeans?

And where's the comfort in emerging from your winter woollies in Spring feeling sluggish and no longer fitting into your jeans?

The sun's out so I want wine

More than one of the people I interviewed for this book told me that as soon as the sun comes out their thoughts turn to pub gardens, chilled bottles of wine and jugs of Pimms. Isn't advertising clever?! When it's Christmas all we see are ads for chocolates, alcohol, Christmas pudding and mince pies, when it's Easter it's all about chocolate eggs and hot cross buns then Summer comes around and every ad break includes reminders of gin and tonics, Pimms and ice cold beers at barbecues.

There are temptations all year round, they just differ from season to season. And resisting the urge to knock back chilled white wine or glasses of Pimms every time the sun comes out requires the same strategies as for any other temptation. What can you do/drink instead? How can you break the chain of events which has you overindulging? Don't deprive yourself totally but if you want to look and feel healthy, sitting in the sun with a chilled glass of wine should be a treat, not a daily event.

See also "I like a drink".

Diets

I've tried to lose weight before and failed

Then this time around take a new approach because, as I've said once already, *if you always do what you've always done you'll always get what you always got.* And that new approach should not involve another Diet.

Here are just a few reasons why Diets will never work for you:

- They are restrictive – and when something is declared off limits, guess what? You can't stop thinking about it. So if your Diet of choice says you can't drink alcohol, and you love a glass of wine, it's not going to make you happy and you are going to struggle to stick to it. The same goes for Diets which ban particular foods or food groups. In the words of one of the dieters I interviewed for this book, "When you're told you can't have things you immediately want them".

- Diets require food intake to be constantly monitored – points, calories, red and green days, etc. So guess what? You end up thinking about food all the time. Not a great idea when you are trying to reduce what you eat.

And that leads on to another problem with Diets: they generally concentrate on reducing food intake, either generally or for certain food groups, so you're constantly feeling deprived.

• Diets also foster self-hatred. When I've interviewed dieters about their experiences they've used words such as "bad" and "naughty" to describe the times they've strayed from their Diet plans, and they regularly feel guilty and angry at themselves. Moreover, as far as I can tell, weight-loss groups with their weekly weigh-ins encourage this judgmental attitude. (For further thoughts on weight-loss groups, see "I'll join a slimming club").

For dieters, all of this gives rise to a pretty difficult relationship with food, and a depressing way to live.

For dieters who manage to stick to their restrictive Diets, it's quite likely that they will lose weight, and some people lose a lot. But they generally mess up their metabolisms so that when they get to the "end" of their Diet, their bodies store fat much more readily, and before too long most people are back where they started. And then they beat themselves up for a lack of willpower and the whole self-hatred thing kicks in.

What I hope you've picked up from all of this is that the problem isn't you – it's the whole concept of Being On A Diet, which is basically a contrived and restricted eating plan with a start and an end date.

In contrast, here's how it works when you're eating healthily:

- It's about *improving the quality* of your food, rather than *reducing the quantity.*

- Eating well is about nurturing your body because you like it and want to take care of it, in contrast to Dieting which seems to be about punishing your body and yourself.

- Healthy eating is a way of life, with no start and end date[3].

- Eating well improves the way your body functions and changes the way it stores or burns fat, so if you do have excess weight to lose, you will lose it.

So what's it to be? Diet or healthy eating?

---

3   I am often reluctant to refer to healthy eating as a Way of Life to new clients with a background of failed diets. The concept of eating differently for the rest of one's life can sound very depressing to someone who sees healthy eating as a form of deprivation. But once my clients start to enjoy the benefits of healthy eating the concept of a lifelong commitment doesn't seem onerous at all.

I'll just crash diet closer to the time

It is possible to lose an impressive amount of weight on a crash diet - *if you stick to it.* In order to lose that impressive amount of weight, you need to follow the diet plan to the letter, which most people will find very difficult. So relying on a last minute crash diet is relying on having the willpower to stick to it.

Also, if you do stick to it, that impressive amount of weight loss is likely to be mainly water. Very restrictive diet plans cause the body to use up its carbohydrate stores, known as glycogen, which is stored with three times its weight in water. When glycogen is lost, the water is lost, hence the weight loss. Now I am not denying that this does bring about a difference in your appearance, but as soon as you start eating normally, your glycogen stores get replenished, as does the water which gets stored with them, and your weight will increase again. So in all honesty, if you wanted to look good for a single day, and you have the dedication to stick to a crash diet, it can help you achieve what you want – temporarily. But this book is about healthy eating, and crash dieting is neither healthy nor a practical long term strategy.

Dieting is too hard

Yes, being on a Diet will be hard. You're following a set of rules devised by someone else, you're restricting your food intake and going without foods you love.

Some Diets will suit you better than others, but generally whichever Diet you choose you're subjecting yourself to a set of contrived rules and often impractical restrictions. And if you're reducing the quantity of your food you're reducing the amount of nutrients

Improve the quality of your food and stop reducing the quantity.

you're getting too. So don't Diet. Improve the quality of your food and stop reducing the quantity.

See "I've tried to lose weight before and failed" for more about this.

I'll join a slimming club

This statement is normally followed by "....because it worked before". So if it worked before, why are you going back?

One of the dieters I interviewed for this book has

signed up with Weight Watchers between 8 and 10 times in her adult life. She was always very successful during the first couple of months and often dropped several stone, but then she'd have a bad week, couldn't face the weigh-in and wouldn't go. She'd tell herself that she'd be extra "good" (note the self-judgmental language) the following week and then go back, but wouldn't manage it, and then dropped out of the group. She'd then try to follow the Weight Watchers Diet on her own, but couldn't manage it, so the following year found herself signing up to the group again. Every time she re-joined she was *a stone heavier* than when she joined up the last time. This is a common pattern with slimming club fans[4] – they are serial joiners. And if they have to go back over and over again, can slimming clubs really be said to work?

The dieter mentioned above didn't only try Weight Watchers. She tried Lighter Life and she lost six stone in three months. In order to achieve that she lived mainly on liquids – shakes, soups, and the occasional food bar. Halfway through her program she was allowed one "normal" meal, and her group leader advised her to have a pint of milk because if she ate real food she "might get the taste for it again". This is the mad, bad reality of weight loss clubs. When she finished the plan,

---

4   *I say "fans" but as no one ever says they enjoy attending slimming clubs perhaps I just mean "regulars".*

our dieter was given advice on "how to start integrating food into her life again". *What?!?!?*

She also told me that she became very, very boring. She was so obsessed with not eating she talked about it all the time. So it wasn't much fun for her but I'm guessing it wasn't much fun for her friends either. And although she did keep the weight off for a while, it did subsequently creep back on, so all that deprivation and misery was for nothing[5].

Moreover, none of the dieters I interviewed who'd attended slimming clubs described the meetings in positive terms. They described weigh-ins as "humiliating", the leaders "patronising" and the general experience "a necessary evil". One dieter said, "By my third attempt at Weight Watchers I was so obsessed with points and food I thought of nothing else". And one dieter told me

Is it time for you to try a different approach?

that she discovered it was perfectly possible to use every one of her Weight Watchers points to eat junk – so even when she stuck to her points allowance she was eating an unhealthy diet completely lacking in nutrients, sending her

5   *I'm pleased to say that this dieter has now lost a significant amount of weight through healthy eating alone – no diet plans, no calorie counting, no liquid meals, no beating herself up if she has a treat. I'd like to claim the credit for coaching her to achieve this but I can't, she's done it alone, and I really enjoyed hearing her story*

blood haywire and giving her constant cravings.

Despite all of this, slimming clubs are still pulling in the business, both at meetings and online. People go back with the view that, "This time I will stick with it", "This time I will make it work". But what's that thing that Einstein said? *Insanity is doing the same thing over and over again and expecting a different result.* Is it time for you to try a different approach?

Dieting is dull

Yes, it is. You're following a restrictive regime, you're having to be constantly vigilant and you're probably thinking about the food you can and can't have all the time. That's really dull, and dull for the people around you if you talk about it all the time.

Also, depending on what you're being told to eat on your Diet, the food itself could be deadly dull – see "Healthy food is boring".

Healthy eating as a lifestyle needn't be dull – invest a little time in finding a range of interesting and nutritious foods which you enjoy and eat them, without counting calories, weighting out portion sizes or totally avoiding certain food groups. Make wise choices in restaurants, have the occasional treat, but eat well because it makes you feel well and because it doesn't feel restrictive or boring.

See also "I've tried to lose weight before and failed".

I've been eating healthily for a week and haven't seen any results

A week is not very long and if you've genuinely made changes to your diet you'll start seeing the benefits over time. If you've been eating badly for years, one good week isn't going to fix it. Nutritional deficiencies are created over months or years, and they will take a while to put right.

If it is weight loss you were hoping for, stick with it. It's going to take time for your hormones to adjust to your new diet and for your body to start processing what you are feeding it in a more efficient way.

I've been eating healthily for a month and haven't seen any results

When nutritional therapist Nick Owen's clients tell him that his recommendations aren't working he asks them to keep a food diary – in photographs. The photographs reveal what his clients aren't telling him, and that usually they aren't following his recommendations as closely as they think.

The photographs often reveal issues with portion sizes. "A little bit" means very different thing to different people. Whilst healthy eating isn't necessarily about reducing quantities, it is about eating an appropriate amount of food.

The photographs also reveal "extras" such as generous dollops of creamy dressings on salad, bread rolls on side plates and grande lattes to accompany healthy meals.

So if you are disappointed that you haven't seen any weight loss, and

Be honest with yourself about how much you're eating.

if you really do have weight to lose, be honest with yourself about how much you're eating, what you're actually putting on your plate, what you might be stealing from your partner's plate and the amount of calories you might be consuming in liquid form such as lattes and smoothies.

But also be patient, because gradual weight loss through improving your diet is likely to be more permanent than weight lost through restricting the quantity of food eaten.

Knowledge

I don't know what I should be eating

It's easy to get confused about what's healthy and what's not, when new and conflicting reports are published daily about what's good to eat, what's not, what will lower your risk of heart disease, what won't, what will cause you to gain weight, what will cause you to lose weight, etc, etc, etc.

A good example of this is the egg. In the 1960s there was a TV advert telling us to "go to work on an egg". Back then it was deemed to be a healthy start to our day. Then in the 1980s we were advised that eggs contain cholesterol which raises cholesterol levels in our bodies so we limited our egg consumption (or ate egg whites only, as we also learnt that all the fat was contained within yolk). But more recently the recommendations have been reversed again – it's now understood that cholesterol in our bodies is not directly caused by cholesterol in food, so eggs are back on the menu, especially the yolks, which are packed full of nutrients.

It's also easy to get confused if you're trying to lose weight and have tried lots of different Diets.

Do you avoid fat, avoid carbohydrates, fast for two days a week, count points, count calories, allow yourself only so many "sins" a week, drink green tea, avoid dairy, etc? Essentially all Diets are about reducing your food intake, so however the Diet is designed, it's really just a means of restricting what you can eat. And Diets are not the same as healthy eating – their objective is quick weight loss, not optimum health.

So if you're feeling confused about what you should be eating, here are two pointers: firstly, don't expect to find advice on healthy eating in the latest Diet book. You're only going to find advice on how to restrict your eating, because that's what Diets do. Secondly, if in doubt, stick to what's close to nature and what hasn't been overly processed. Go for unprocessed, natural food and you can't go far wrong.

If in doubt, stick to what's close to nature.

I don't know what I shouldn't be eating

There are some things we all know are bad for us – overly processed foods, sugary foods, supersize portions, eating out of boredom rather than hunger, too much alcohol. If you avoid all of those, you're already well on the way to eating well. But clever marketing has persuaded us that some foods are healthy when they are not. Fruit juices, cereals and cereal bars, breakfast biscuits, sports drinks and ready meals are all present-ed to us with descriptions designed to have us believe that they are good for us – "one of your five a day", "whole grain", "a source of fibre", "added vitamins", "low in fat". In fact all of these foods are processed, and processing depletes nutrients. That orange juice containing "one of your five a day" is likely to have been pasteurised and stripped of most of the nutritional benefits you'd get from an orange in its natural form. Those breakfast biscuits could well be made of whole grains, but those grains are processed and broken down into sugars. That ready meal that's low in fat is probably also low in vitamins and fibre and high in sugar.

So if it's processed, if it includes ingredients you don't recognise or ingredients which don't resemble their natural form, you probably shouldn't be eating it.

And if you're looking at something in a wrapper which tells you, "Enjoy as part of a balanced diet" you are definitely looking at something unhealthy. What that message is actually saying is, "If you eat this, you're going to have to make sure the rest of food you eat is going to nourish you, because this won't".

I can't cook

Nobody can when they start out. But you don't need to be a great cook to prepare healthy food. Remember healthy food is all about fresh, natural ingredients, so the less you do to those ingredients, the better.

All of the following require very little skill:

- Roasting, grilling, pan frying, barbecuing meat
- Roasting, grilling, barbecuing, steaming vegetables
- Assembling a salad
- Poaching, frying, scrambling or boiling eggs
- Baking a sweet potato in its jacket
- Casseroling or stewing meat and/or vegetables
- Stir frying meat and/or vegetables

And most of these ideas also require very little time – probably about as much time as you'd spend watching a ready meal revolve in a microwave.

I don't know what to cook

You've been shopping and your fridge is full of fresh, nutritious foods. And you're standing looking at them and haven't a clue what to do with them.

Before you go shopping do you have a plan? Planning always helps. Make a list of the meals you'd like to cook and then list the ingredients you'll need. That's your shopping list. If you don't do this you could well end up with a random selection of foods and no idea what to do with them.

So do a bit of research into new recipes, and plan your shopping around them – this also means you'll avoid having lots of food you don't need in the house.

See also "I'm too stressed to think about cooking something healthy".

Body

I'm starving

Are you? Really? You could just be bored. At times, for want of anything interesting to do, people snack. It could be a sugar craving, caused by a blood sugar dip caused in turn by a high carbohydrate meal a short time ago.

You could just be thirsty. If you're dehydrated, you'll be tired, and you could mistake that feeling for hunger. It could just be meal time. If you have lunch or dinner at a particular time each day, you're going to be programmed to expect food at that time.

So how can you tell if you are really hungry? Have a glass of water first, and wait a few minutes – you've got nothing to lose except possibly that "hunger".

If you're still hungry after a few minutes, what are you hungry for? If it's chocolate, pizza or some other high-calorie or high-sugar food, you could well be suffering from unstable blood sugar. And if it's meal time, fine, go ahead and eat, make it healthy and acknowledge that claiming to be "starving" might be a slight exaggeration!

See also "I get cravings".

I'm too tired to think about preparing healthy food

You get home from work, you're tired, you've been planning to prepare something healthy, but the thought of standing in the kitchen chopping vegetables and then waiting for them to cook just fills you with dread. So what do you do? Order a takeaway, open a packet of biscuits, eat several packets of crisps?

It doesn't have to follow that just because you don't want to spend time preparing a nutritious meal that you have to go to the other extreme. It needn't be so black and white. If you own a freezer and a microwave you could have prepared a stash of healthy frozen meals for moments like this. Or you could have an apple and some nut butter, some crudités and houmous, some cold meats and salad, boiled eggs...there are lots of things you can keep in your fridge or kitchen cupboard which take only a couple of minutes to prepare.

Being too tired to prepare a healthy meal does not mean that what you do eat has to be processed junk food. (And that wouldn't be an option anyway if you didn't have it in the house).

See also "I'm too stressed to think about cooking something healthy" – particularly if you've ever made yourself a fish finger sandwich!

It's my age

It's generally accepted that as we get older we get fatter. It's said to be partly to do with becoming less active as we age, but we also undergo hormonal changes which affect how our bodies maintain muscle and store fat.

But we probably overestimate the effect of ageing, particularly up to our 50s. It's not just age. A lifetime of yoyo dieting can result in a damaged metabolism (which can be remedied by improving your diet now). Retirement or your kids leaving home could result in more leisure time and/or disposable income, leading to more eating out, more holidays or more socialising and alcohol. Those things will all have an effect on your health and weight regardless of age.

It's not a given that as you age your health is destined to deteriorate.

I am a good example of how it's possible for your health to improve as you get older. I am close to 50 and I am leaner and healthier than I was in my 20s and 30s. Because back then I had a terrible diet and drank way too much wine. So it's not a given that as you age your health is destined to deteriorate. Lifestyle has a *big* part to play.

And even if we accept that weight loss does become harder as we age, that doesn't mean you can't still be healthy. Forgetting weight loss totally, eating well will still give you all the other health benefits, and ward off diet-related diseases such as diabetes, whether you're 20 or 70.

I'm feeling ill

Poor you. If you're feeling rough and sorry for yourself then having a treat to cheer yourself up won't hurt. But note that was "treat" in the singular, not the plural! There's a big difference between having a portion of something you really enjoy to cheer yourself up and abandoning all attempts to eat well until you're fully recovered.

If you're under the weather then healthy food is just what your body needs to aid its recovery, so try to view eating while you're ill as something you are doing to nurture yourself rather than comfort yourself.

It's my hormones

One of the people I spoke to when researching for this book told me that she eats really well for three weeks every month but said that in the week running up to her period it "all goes wrong".

It's a fact that women's hormones can go haywire at this time, and it's generally accepted that this causes sugar cravings, binge eating and unwise food choices. Cortisol and serotonin levels can go out of balance and body temperature can rise, all of which can cause low energy levels and increased appetite.

However, the women I spoke to about this said the following:

"I know I am going to be bloated anyway so I think I may as well have chocolate"

"I tell myself when I am feeling like this I need sugar"

"I know it's that time and I know I am going to want chocolate"

None of these comments relate to a physical compulsion to eat more. Instead they reveal *expectations* about wanting to eat more, and although your body could well feel different in the run up to your period, it will definitely feel different if that's your expectation. So do ask yourself if you are actually at the mercy of your hormones or whether you are telling yourself you'll feel different in order to give yourself permission to eat what you know you shouldn't.

Finally, good nutrition does significantly reduce pre-menstrual symptoms and food cravings. One of my clients told me that before she changed her eating habits she would have intense cravings for sugar just before her period. She'd go out and buy three Snickers bars at once, eat them all, and then crave more. Now, after cleaning up her diet and cutting out sugars, she has *no cravings at all*. So pre-menstrual cravings are not an excuse to eat badly, but a reason to eat as well as possible!

I am already thin so don't need to eat healthily

If your only goal is to be thin, then yes, strictly speaking you don't need to eat healthily.

You can be very thin but live on a diet of coffee, cigarettes and chocolate. I know someone who really did exist on those three things, and she was thin but she was also always ill. Her employer's HR manager had to have a word with her about the amount of time she took off sick. And she always looked absolutely dreadful.

Bodies are meant to be well nourished.

Bodies are meant to be well nourished – if yours is not, you run the risk of feeling tired all the time, catching lots of colds, getting lectures from your doctor about high cholesterol and blood sugar readings and looking generally below par. So even if you are thin, you still need to take care of yourself. Healthy eating is not the same as being on a Diet, and healthy eating is not about losing weight. It's about nourishing your body so that you can enjoy life.

My partner/friends say I will get too thin

You won't get too thin if you eat enough!

All of my family struggle with their weight

What families share as well as genetics is eating habits. Children learn to how to eat from their parents. So do you struggle with your weight because of genetics or because of how you have learnt to eat?

Well, does it really matter? Because you can't

change your genetics, but you can change how you eat. And even if you believe that you are unlucky genetically, it doesn't mean that changing your diet won't have a positive effect.

Do you eat over-sized portions? Do you have a handful of biscuits every time you have a cup of tea? Do you always have a snack you don't need before you go to bed? Do you always clear your plate? Have you never developed a taste for vegetables? Do you reward yourself with bars of chocolate? Do you always have to have something sweet to finish off a meal? Is a meal not a meal without chips? All of these are things which clients have told me that they learnt from their parents and carried forward into adulthood. And all of these behaviours can be changed.

So before you tell yourself that you can't change your genetics, ask yourself what can you change?

Social Life

I like a drink

Alcohol will always do damage to your healthy eating goals. It prevents your body's organs from working as they should and it's a nutrient sapper. It inhibits your body's usual fat burning processes and dehydrates you so that your skin looks dull and your energy levels plummet. You'll never feel or look great if you drink a lot.

I like a drink too – in fact in my earlier years I *loved* drinking. I exercised regularly and ate relatively well but I was never as energetic, lean or healthy looking as I wanted to be. No one ever told me I looked well, in fact people would often tell me I looked tired, and that's because I did. The alcohol was sabotaging all the other efforts I was making. I got fed up of not looking fit or toned when I was in the gym four or five times a week, and eventually I had to acknowledge that that wouldn't change while I was drinking so much wine. I had to make a decision – make the workouts as effective as possible by reducing the amount of alcohol I consumed or resign myself to never feeling as great as I wanted to feel. And that's the deal – if you want to feel energetic, alert, glowing, lean and well, you can't indulge your love of wine or beer *all of the time.* There's no need for total abstinence, but you'll need to start experimenting with reductions in frequency and amounts until you find a way of drinking which doesn't hamper your efforts to feel and look better.

So how to reduce the amount you drink? If you have a ready supply of alcohol in the house, you'll be constantly tempted, so consider getting rid of it (preferably not all in one sitting). See "I've got no willpower" for more thoughts on dealing with temptation.

If you like visits to the pub, could you turn up later so there's less drinking time? Or do something else with some of your evenings?

And think of the money you could save if you're not forking out for bottles of wine, overpriced cocktails and rounds in the pub – what non-food treats could you buy instead as a reward for yourself?

The other downside of alcohol is that it weakens your resolve to eat well - see "I'm drunk".

My partner ordered a takeaway

Just because your partner orders a takeaway doesn't mean you have to join him/her, but I accept that sitting in the same room as someone enjoying a feast could be pretty grim if you're abstaining.

So you're trying to eat healthily but your partner wants a takeaway, and because you want to eat together you go along with the idea and make your choice.

I'm not going to name the healthiest options on each type of takeaway menu here, but they are there, and I am guessing you *know* what the healthiest options are. It's just that you haven't chosen them. For a lot of people takeaways trigger this thought: "Well it's not going to be a perfect meal so I may as well just order all the unhealthiest items on the menu, and while I'm at it I'll order far more than I need". So the healthier options don't get a look in.

> It's no treat to feel overly full, sluggish and angry at yourself afterwards.

Takeaways are a treat, but by making clever choices you don't have to completely sabotage your efforts to eat well. It's no treat to feel overly full, sluggish and angry at yourself afterwards. Pick out those healthier options and give them a go.

See also "I'm eating out".

It's the weekend

"Hooray it's the weekend, forget all that healthy eating stuff, let's go mad with booze and food". Most people don't say that out loud but their actions reveal that that's what they are thinking.

Yes, you've had a busy week at work and you've eaten well all week. Yes, the weekend is a time to chill out, do the things you enjoy and be happy. But how happy are you going to be on Monday morning when you're feeling less than your best because of a weekend of high-calorie foods and too much alcohol?

When Nick Owen's clients ask him about how much they can get away with at the weekend, he sketches a flight of stairs for them. He explains that eating well all week will take them up quite a few of the steps. But then he shows them that an overindulgent weekend will take them back down a few again. Nick then asks, "How many steps are you willing to go back down again each weekend?"

See also "I'll start again on Monday".

I'm eating out

A couple of my interviewees told me that when they eat

out they would never consider searching out the healthier options on the menu. One of them said, "If I'm going out I want to enjoy it". The implication being: forget enjoying the company of the people you're with, forget about soaking up the atmosphere, it's all about the food.

Do you see eating out as a break from "normal" eating? It's not, it's still just choosing food and feeding your body. Your body doesn't process the food eaten in restaurants any differently to the food you eat at home.

Your body doesn't process the food eaten in restaurants any differently to the food you eat at home.

So whilst you might not want to abstain totally from all the goodies on offer, you don't have to have e*verything* you like. You don't have to have several pieces of bread from the bread basket before the starter has arrived, you don't have to choose three unhealthy courses, you don't have to order a side dish of fries to accompany a generously sized main course, you don't have to steal fries off your partner's plate, you don't have to eat everything on your plate(s) once you're full.

Instead, try reaching a compromise with yourself. If you want a burger, have it without the bun, ask for salad instead of fries, or share a portion of fries. If you want a dessert, don't have a starter. If you want a stodgy main course have a salad for starter. Make *some* healthy choices to give yourself permission to enjoy an unhealthy one. It doesn't have to be all or nothing.

And don't be afraid to ask for a variation on whatever's listed on the menu – you're the paying

> It doesn't have to be all or nothing.

customer and restaurants should be happy to accommodate you - salad with dressing on the side, steak without sauce, dessert without extra cream?

I'm drunk

Alcohol changes what's going on inside your body, so that your organs and chemical/hormonal processes are diverted from doing all the things they're supposed to be doing in order to rid your body of the alcohol as soon as possible. While your body is dealing with alcohol it's not burning fat nor using the energy from the food you've been eating in the most efficient way. In fact your body will be in fat storage mode.

On top of this, alcohol weakens resolve, so at the very worst time possible to be eating crisps, bowls of chips, bar snacks and kebabs on the way home, you're actually really likely to do so.

What's the solution? Well, at least be extremely mindful of the fact that anything consumed while your body is processing an onslaught of alcohol is far more likely to be turned into fat than at other times. It might not always stop you but it could at least give you pause for thought. And since alcohol saps nutrients, the more nutritious the meal, the less the nutrient deficit you'll suffer overall. Not easy things to keep in mind if you're totally plastered, but before you go out try to eat something healthy[6], which might help to allay the effects of what you do drink, and if you don't go mad with the drinks you might just manage to keep your focus on what matters most – that is a healthy, energetic and happy you, not rubbish bar snacks and fast food!

See also "I like a drink".

I'm hungover

Ok, so you got legless last night. You're dehydrated, low in mental and physical energy and you just want a quick fix. Bacon sandwich on white bread, anybody? A trip to McDonalds, a triple chocolate muffin, a full sugar Coke or a Red Bull? These are hardly going to help

6   *That doesn't mean stodge to "soak up the alcohol" as many people believe – something protein based is far better*

replenish your lost nutrients, nor will they provide sustained energy. At best they'll be temporarily comforting and then you'll return to feeling just as bad as before. And you'll just be prolonging the period of unhealthy eating which started last night.

Try to choose foods which will aid your recovery by restoring depleted nutrients. What is the most nutritious thing you can prepare and feed your body right now?

And don't forget that drinking lots of water and getting some extra sleep will do more to make you feel better than any amount of processed and sugary foods.

See also "I'm feeling ill".

It would be rude to say no

When you're invited round to someone's house it's usual to find food on offer when you get there – if you're going over for coffee there'll be biscuits and/or cake, if you're going over for drinks there'll be nibbles, and if you're invited for dinner, well, there will probably be much more food on offer than you normally eat in one sitting. It's all part of being hospitable. And when someone has bought and prepared this food for you, it feels ungrateful to refuse.

Ideally of course all of your friends would be as

focused on healthy eating as you are, and be serving up nutritious snacks and meals when they invite you round, but that's not always going to be the case. So what do you do if you're offered biscuits, cakes, or a second helping of someone's homemade pie or dessert? How can you say no without offending?

Work on polite refusals.

What reason could you give which, even if it wasn't *quite* true, might make you feel more comfortable about saying no to plates of cakes and biscuits? Work on polite refusals such as, "No thanks, I had a big lunch and I am still full", "No thanks, I'm going out for lunch/dinner and want to save myself", "No thanks, I had something to eat before I came here".

When you're invited to dinner, if you don't want to eat everything that's put in front of you, try, "No thanks, that was lovely but I can't eat another mouthful". Think up some of your own polite refusals and practice saying these before you go so they're ready to trip off your tongue when you arrive.

And if you're being invited to dinner, can you offer to take a dessert, and make it a healthy one?

Of course if it's a special occasion then don't be too hard on yourself if you want to enjoy what's on offer, but even then don't feel obliged to accept food you don't want to eat just to be polite. Put your healthy eating goals first, and have your polite refusal at the ready.

See also "My friends talked me into it" if your friends won't take no for an answer.

It's Christmas/Easter/my birthday

If it's your birthday, go for it, have a treat – it's *your birthday!* And if it's Christmas Day or Easter Sunday, then it's just one day, so again, go on, have a treat, these days only come around once a year.

But if it's just December, or the week running up to Easter, read on.

Last November I walked into a coffee shop and I was offered samples of their new Christmas menu – seven weeks before Christmas. Our local café started selling mince pies in late November and I've had been to Christmas parties as early as December 4th. And that's the problem with Christmas – it starts too early. If you work in an office there'll be more than the usual number of cakes, chocolates and treats sitting around, perhaps donated by grateful clients or bosses in a festive mood. And you're likely to be socialising a whole lot more. The same goes for Easter – people start bringing chocolate eggs and hot cross buns into the office at least a week before the actual event.

There is a big difference between allowing yourself a few treats at Christmas and relaxing as soon as you see your first Christmas tree and then staying relaxed until January 1st! Keep this at the forefront of your mind as the festive season kicks in. Ask yourself each time you're offered a cheese straw, slice of cake, mince pie, a handful of chocolates, etc – *is it actually Christmas yet?!* And promise yourself that when it really is Christmas (Christmas Eve, Christmas Day, Boxing Day), you can have the treats.

I have to entertain clients

This can be tricky – if you're entertaining someone on whom your livelihood or employer's profits depend, you're beholden to keep them happy. You might also have a boss who expects you to go out and match the clients drink for drink. I appreciate it can be difficult to simply say you won't be drinking, as I have had this responsibility in the past when I had a client-facing job. I have a couple of suggestions – if you're asked in advance by your boss whether you can entertain someone one evening in the future, say you're busy that evening.

And if you can't wriggle out of it say you're on painkillers or some other sort of pills which means you can't drink, or can't drink very much. Or could you arrange to drive home, or at least say you have to? This does of course depend on your attitude to white lies, but all it takes is one little white lie at the start of the evening and then you're committed.

And if you're trying to cut down on drinking in general, ask yourself this: when you do have a precious drink, do you really want it to be with a client or would you rather save the treat to share with someone with whom you really enjoy spending time?

See also "I'm eating out".

My friends talked me into it

What is it about some people that they can't accept it when you say, "No thanks, not for me?"

I've been there – "No thanks, I'm trying to cut down on sugar", or back in the days when I thought Dieting was a good idea, "No thanks, I'm on a diet". Saying no when someone else is saying yes does seem to bring out the need in people to attempt to get you to join them in their indulgence (and this does only tend to occur when *they* are indulging). It probably says more about how they feel about their own indulgence than it does about what they think about you, but since you can't change other people, what can you do to avoid giving in just to shut them up?

Well, in my experience, the more positive you make your reason, the more likely people are to accept it. So, I've learned that when I go to the pub and don't intend to drink, I give a positive reason for not drinking rather than a reason relating to deprivation: "I'm not drinking tonight as I am looking forward to feeling good for my day out tomorrow" rather than, "I've been drinking too much this month and I am trying to cut down". Not sure why it works, but it does.

So the next time someone is passing cakes around the office and you don't want one, start with a simple, "No, thanks". Then if that's not accepted, tell them you're still full from your last meal, or you're saving yourself for a fantastic meal that evening, or you've got something in your bag that you'd prefer to eat instead. Anything, as long as it's stated in the positive. And if it's not entirely true, well, does it matter if you achieve the desired effect?

Finances

Healthy food is expensive

Yes, quality, fresh, natural food is more expensive than processed food. But it's also much higher in nutrients. So on balance you're getting more for your money with healthy purchases.

Every time you choose to eat something fresh and natural instead of something processed you are investing in your health. So consider money spent on good food as an investment in your future self – a healthy and happy you.

Then, when you find yourself hesitating over the cost of an item of food in the supermarket, ask yourself what else would you spend that amount of money on, without even thinking? Let's say it's £4.00 – that's about the same price as a coffee and a muffin on the way to work in the morning or a glossy magazine, and it's probably less than the last new nail varnish or lipstick you bought on a whim, or that cocktail you ordered in a restaurant whilst waiting for your meal just because it was on promotion. Have a think about your spending priorities, and about which purchases will actually be most effective in making you feel better about yourself.

One final thought – the most expensive food is the food which gets thrown away at the end of the week because it's past its best. So make sure you cook and eat all of the healthy food you buy!

It was two for the price of one

But did you need two? In fact, if we're talking about processed food which is devoid of nutrients and/or full of sugar, did you even need one?

If you eat the two so as not to waste them, see "I don't like leaving leftovers".

Location

I'm on holiday

A holiday is a chance to take a break from the usual pressures and pains of your working life, to relax and to feel good about yourself. And that's likely to include having a few drinks, enjoying meals out and trying out new foods. It would be a pretty dull holiday if you didn't allow yourself any of these things.

Don't return home having undone all of your good work.

But this is no reason to go to extremes – your body still has the same nutritional requirements whether you're on holiday or at home, so don't abandon all attempts to eat healthily. Decide on a few things you can still do while you're away – for instance, eat all of your five a day, avoid white bread, eat some good fats (oily fish, olive oil, nuts). You can combine lots of healthy habits with a few treats so that you don't return home having undone all of the good work you did before you went away.

See "It's the weekend" and ask yourself how far back down the flight of stairs you're willing to go.

I'm travelling for work

I had to travel from London up to Manchester last week, and while I stood on the concourse waiting for my train at 7.30 in the morning I took a look around at the food on offer: sausage baguettes, muffins, croissants, pretzels, pastries, Cornish pasties and cookies. Then when I got on the train I went to the buffet to buy some water and was confronted with shelves full of crisps, sausage rolls, unappetising sandwiches made with poor quality bread and minimal filling, biscuits, chocolate, sugary drinks, wine and beer. It's as if train operators have all got together and hatched a plan to make their customers eat as much junk as possible.

If you're travelling around by car it's no better – stop off at a motorway service station and you're confronted by chocolate bars at the till and if you're looking for lunch it's going to be a choice between a burger and fries, a pre-packed poor quality sandwich or panini, crisps or cakes.

When you arrive at your destination you might find yourself at the mercy of a staff canteen or a sandwich van, and then on your journey home you run the gauntlet of a motorway service station or a train station all over again.

This is all pretty depressing, as there really is very little opportunity to make good food choices on the go.

So your best option is to take your food with you. Take breakfast if you don't eat before you go out, and take lunch and snacks. Take too many, just in case you're de-layed and out for longer than you expect. Don't leave yourself in the posi-tion where you find your-self without food and so hungry that you resort to buying over-priced, over-pro-cessed food which you don't really enjoy and won't do you any good.

Your best option is to take your food with you.

If you're travelling abroad, you'll have the added challenges of airports, planes and hotels. Airports of-fer a similar set of choices to train stations and motor-way service stations, and there's nothing positive to say about the food you're likely to get on the plane. Once again, take your own food for the journey. Even if it's not quite as healthy as a meal you could prepare in your own kitchen, it's ten times better than the food on sale as you travel.

If you're staying and eating in a hotel, treat your meal like any restaurant meal and don't be afraid to go "off-menu" – ask the server for salad or vegetables rather than fries, sauce or dressing on the side, or the burger without the bun. See also "I'm eating out".

Logistics

I didn't have any healthy food in the house

Why not, when your goal is to be eating healthy food?!

The more you plan, the more successful you'll be in achieving your goals, as you can look ahead to possible obstacles and problems and put measures in place to overcome them. So you can solve this one with some forward planning. For instance, if you know that next week it's likely you're going to have to work late and by the time you get home the supermarket will be closed and you won't be able to buy food, buy something in advance to keep in the freezer ready for that eventuality.

Set aside some time every week to review what you've got in the house and what you might need for the coming week. If you've got three evenings at home, plan for four meals, so you've got contingency in case one of your evenings out is cancelled. If you're going to be at home during the day, plan for lunches and snacks too. It sounds obvious, but if you're at home, hungry, and looking at an empty fridge, or a cupboard only stocked with biscuits and crisps, you've not been doing enough planning!

See also "I don't have the time to shop for healthy food".

I'm surrounded by treats at work

When I worked in an office I was often surrounded by treats at work. Or at least they were someone's idea of a treat, but not necessarily my idea of one. So yes you might be surrounded by chocolates and biscuits and cakes, but ask yourself this: if you were choosing to buy yourself a treat, is this exactly what you'd have? Because if it's not, why eat it now? If you're going to have a treat, shouldn't it be something you'll really love? Why waste the calories on something you wouldn't normally choose for yourself, just because it's there?

Wait, and buy yourself your favourite type of chocolate or cake or have a glass of your favourite wine instead, which you can truly savour and enjoy, instead of just eating things you feel indifferent about just because they're there and they're free.

See also "It's Christmas/Easter/my birthday".

Healthy eating doesn't fit in with my routine

I often hear people say that they don't have the opportunity to organise healthy food for themselves - they say they can't search out healthy snacks on the go, or there's nowhere to assemble a salad at work, or they can't fit regular meals into their routine.

I asked Nick Owen to tell me one key thing which his clients could do to make healthy eating work for them and without hesitation he said, "Use their imagination". He told me that often people allow themselves to fall at the first hurdle because they aren't being creative. So someone says she can't take a salad to work because preparing, transporting and then eating it is too messy, but this is because she's thinking of how she'd prepare a salad at home – sliced tomatoes, grated carrot, etc and dressing. But she could take cherry tomatoes and carrot sticks with a dip. Same components, no mess. Someone else says that eating fruit on the go is too messy, based on his experience of eating big juicy oranges at home. But how about a handful of grapes, an apple or a couple of satsumas instead? Lots of fruit is perfectly portable.

In terms of fitting food into your routine, if you're fitting shopping, preparing and eating unhealthy food into your current day, you've got the time to fit in healthy food instead. It takes no longer to shop for healthy food, and it doesn't have to take longer to prepare or eat it if you make clever choices.

If your days are so hectic that you go for hours without eating, be imaginative about making time. Make an appointment with yourself to eat, and plan your other commitments around it. If you're employed, everyone is entitled to a break during the working day, and why put your employer's profits above your own health? If you're self-employed, then you have the freedom to take a break whenever you want – use this freedom, it's a privilege. You only need a few minutes to eat a snack. If that means you leave the office a few minutes later in the evening, you'll be leaving it better nourished.

> Make an appointment with yourself to eat, and plan your other commitments around it.

What this really boils down to is the old saying, "Where there's a will there's a way". If you really want to clean up your diet, eat regular meals and reap the benefits, you can use your imagination and make some changes to your routine to do so.

I forgot to bring my healthy lunch into the office

It's probably too late to fix this this time around, but what can you to ensure it doesn't happen again? When you fly off on holiday, do you ever forget your passport? Or the last time you had tickets for a gig did you leave them on the kitchen table when you left the house? I am guessing not. Those things were so important to you that you made sure you remembered to take them with you – perhaps you stuck a "don't forget…" post-it note on your fridge, or put a reminder on your iPhone, or located your passport a few days before and put it somewhere close to hand. Do you do any of these things to remind you to take your lunch with you?

Or how about a contingency plan? Can you take an extra lunch in at the start of the week to keep in the fridge at work, so that if you do forget later in the week you've got an alternative?

If you care enough about something you will ensure that everything is in place to make it happen.

Time

I'm too busy to prepare healthy food

Marketing has a lot to answer for. Food is advertised as "Ready in a few minutes", "Great for busy mums", "For time-pressured people", "For snacking on the go". The implication is that we are all too busy to prepare and sit down to eat real food, and we must believe it, based on the number of cabinets dedicated to ready meals in supermarkets these days.

Fetch a piece of paper and a pen. Write down how you spend a typical day – getting up, showering, watching TV, checking Facebook and Instagram, chatting, reading magazines, painting your nails, gaming…..? Then take a look at your list and tell me whether every activity you've written down is a productive one.

Healthy food doesn't take hours to prepare. It can take a few minutes – you could assemble a salad, grill some meat, create a stir fry, make an omelette or scramble some eggs. Or heat up a portion of something wholesome you've prepared in advance and frozen. None of those things will take much longer than the time you spend watching a ready meal rotating in a microwave.

Also, remind yourself that even healthy-sounding ready meals are never going to be nutritious. A dish of "prime beef with country garden vegetables" is going to be made with poor cuts of meat and processed vegetables with depleted nutrients. And a calorie counted, low fat, or "lite" ready meal is very unlikely to be a healthy option – remember that healthy eating is not about how few calories you eat, it's about the amount of nutrients to be found in your food.

Make sure you've got the necessary ingredients in the house for quick, nutritious meals – see "I didn't have any healthy food in the house" for more on the importance of planning.

See also "I'm too stressed to think about healthy food".

I don't have the time to shop for healthy food

Then don't – do it online and get it delivered. This excuse might have been more valid ten years ago before the rise of mini supermarkets and delivery services, but now if you've got access to the internet you can have anything delivered to your house. All you have to do is to be in when it arrives.

The Lamest Excuses of All

I hate cottage cheese

Then don't eat it.

I don't like tinned tuna, tomatoes or bananas. So I don't eat them. But that doesn't stop me having a healthy diet. There are hundreds of other foods which are healthy and tasty to enjoy. It's not all about cottage cheese.

See also "Healthy food is boring" – it doesn't have to be!

I'm starting a diet tomorrow so I may as well pig out tonight

When you start your new regime tomorrow you'll have a certain amount of body fat to lose. If you pig out now, you're increasing that amount. Why make it harder for yourself?

If you're saying this I'm guessing you view Diets as

finite projects with start and end dates. So when you are Not On A Diet you overindulge and make poor food choices. But this just makes the Diet you are starting tomorrow harder, and more likely to fail, which will repeat the cycle all over again. Doesn't make a lot of sense, does it?

> Eating healthily shouldn't have an on/off switch.

Eating healthily shouldn't have an on/off switch. If you're kind to yourself and stop subjecting yourself to punishing periods of deprivation and restricted food intake, and instead nurture your body with appropriate quantities of good food and occasional treats, you shouldn't feel the need to go Off Diet, as you'll never be on one. Nor will you find yourself eating as much junk food as you can the day before a Diet because you are dreading the deprivation.

I'm eating out tonight

Each day doesn't have to be an all or nothing attempt at eating healthily. So what if you're going out tonight? It doesn't mean that the day is necessarily ruined, particularly if you don't assume that your only option is to eat badly when you're out (see "I'm eating out").

If you eat well all day and make clever choices from the menu when you're out, you will have had a healthy day and you'll feel great tomorrow.

If you eat well all day and then make poor choices from the menu when you're out, you won't have had a perfect day but you won't have had a disastrous day either and you can move on from it tomorrow.

If you eat badly all day and then make poor choices from the menu when you're out, how are you going to feel tomorrow?

I've eaten well all week

So you're going to undo it all now?

As I keep saying, everyone should have a treat occasionally, and if you save your treats for the weekend, then go ahead, just make sure it's something you really love and take the time to savour it.

But if you're about to give yourself permission to forget all about eating well until Monday, take a look at "It's the weekend" and ask yourself how many steps are you willing to go back down each weekend?

I've messed up so I will start again tomorrow/on Monday

One muffin or bar of chocolate is not going to undo several days of healthy eating, but so many of my clients see one slip up as a complete failure.

Think of healthy eating as something you need to do 80-90% of the time. The remaining percentage is yours to use how you like. So if it's Wednesday, and you eat four meals a day which up until now have been healthy, and you're beating yourself up because you've had a takeaway pizza for dinner consider this: that's just one twelfth of the meals you've eaten so far this week.

Your diet does not have to be perfect.

That works out at 8.5% of your meals. So 91.5% of your meals have been nutritious ones. Not bad going, and certainly no reason whatsoever to abandon all attempts to eat well for the rest of the week.

Your diet does not have to be perfect. So don't beat yourself up if it's not, and don't punish yourself further by eating junk for the rest of the week. The key to having a healthy diet is not letting one sub-standard meal trip you up, and to get back to eating the good stuff immediately afterwards.

I deserved a treat

You're not a dog!

Some Final Thoughts

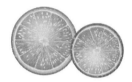

You'll never regret a healthy meal. Every decision you make to choose nutritious, natural foods instead of processed, sugary, nutritionally empty foods is one step closer to a more energetic, happy, healthy you.

And once you've experienced feeling good, looking good, having lots of energy and feeling well (and everything else you have on your Benefits List), you'll never want to go back to eating the foods which made feel you feel less than your best.

But if you've spent years eating processed, sugary, nutrient depleted foods, and if you've ever been on a weight-loss Diet, developing a better relationship with food will take time.

So here are some final thoughts for you to take away with you:

Healthy eating doesn't have to have an on/off switch.

Don't abandon all efforts to eat well for another day/week just because you've succumbed to one doughnut. In the grand scheme of things one doughnut is not a major disaster. Move on and *don't beat yourself up.* Guilt achieves nothing.

Plan, plan plan!

Without planning, things go awry. Plan meals in advance, make food shopping lists and carry healthy snacks with you when you are travelling around so that you don't find yourself at the mercy of fast food shops. The amount of planning you do will have a direct effect on the likelihood of success.

You don't have to be perfect

Nick Owen says, "100% perfect eating is no good for anyone". He tells a story of a client who said she'd told all of her friends and colleagues how committed she was to eating healthily to lose weight and that she didn't want them to tempt her with treats or opportunities for overindulging. And she kept telling them. When Nick saw her again and asked her how it was going she said, "I'm not eating out much now as my friends don't invite me anymore" – it's dull trying to be perfect but it's also dull for those around you if you are constantly talking about it and turning down every opportunity for enjoyment. Pleasure is a nutrient, and it's good for us, so if you love pizza, have one once in a while.

Aim for 80-90% quality food

Use the remaining percentage to have something you really enjoy – but do make sure it's something you *really* enjoy, and savour it. Make the absolute most of the moment.

Be willing to learn and be open to new ideas

If you've lived on low calorie ready meals, fast food and sugary drinks or followed Diet rules for years, accept that you aren't necessarily equipped with the knowledge to make the best food choices. Read up on healthy eating and get advice from professionals. And be willing to try what they suggest, even if it goes against what you've believed so far, or even if it involves new foods that you're not sure you'll like. Be open-minded and give things a chance.

Mind your language

Speak about healthy eating in the positive. Don't speak about what you're giving up or what you want to change about yourself – talk instead of the benefits you are looking forward to and how your new way of eating is going to make you feel, or is making you feel already. So instead of saying, "I can't have a baguette for lunch as I'm banned from eating white carbs", try saying something like, "I prefer to have a salad for lunch, I find it makes me feel much more alert in the afternoon". You're not depriving yourself, you're making a positive choice.

Give yourself time to develop new habits

Bad habits take a while to break but good habits take equally long to form, so give yourself plenty of time. Don't aim to make one great big change. Lots of small changes which stick, built up gradually, are much more effective than a great big change that you can't maintain. And two steps forward, one step back is still forward movement over all.

Many nutrition experts will tell you that healthy eating has to be a Way of Life, but I believe that the concept of eating differently for the rest of your life can sound really depressing if you've struggled for years with food and Diets. Anyone with a history of Dieting tends to see healthy eating as a form of deprivation, so turning that into a lifelong commitment is going to sound pretty unappealing. Who would want a lifetime of deprivation?! But by making slow, gradual changes to your diet you will begin to experience the positive aspects of healthy eating and find that they outweigh any negatives. You'll find that healthy food doesn't have to be boring, you don't have to be 100% perfect, it's not about eating less and that you can ditch the guilt over the odd slip-up. Then the concept of that lifelong commitment won't seem so tough. In fact it will get easier and easier, because it feels so good.

So there you have it – how healthy eating doesn't

have to be difficult and how you can make healthy habits stick. Start changing your relationship with food and you'll change your relationship with your body – you'll be feeding and nourishing it because you love it, not depriving it and punishing it because you hate it. It will pay you back big time.

And no more excuses!

I'd love to hear from you if this book has helped you – or if you have an excuse which I have missed! Email me at joanne@joannehenson.co.uk

Acknowledgements

I'd like to say a big thank you to the following individuals:

Nutritional therapist Nick Owen (what-food.co.uk) for his valuable insights into why people choose to change their eating habits and what they most struggle with

Paula Kirby and Andy Sutton for their proof reading skills and their feedback on my first draft

Susan Green for her insights into why our relationship with food can be so fraught with difficulty and her frank and revealing stories about slimming clubs

Denise Neary and Paula Kirby (again!) for their entertaining stories of the highs and lows of Dieting

Kay Henson for filling in some big gaps and giving me her own ideas and stories

Duda Jadrijevic for her insights into hormonal eating

Reference/
Bibliography

Charlotte Watts, The Top 100 Recipes for Happy Kids:
Keep Your Child Alert, Focused and Active
Duncan Baird, 2007

Anita Bean, Healthy Eating for Kids
A & C Black, 2007

Index

Also in this series

What's Your Excuse for not Getting Fit?

Joanne Henson
Overcome your excuses and get active, healthy and happy

Do you want to be fit, lean and healthy, but find that all too often life gets in the way? Do you own a gym membership you don't use, or take up running every January only to give up in February? Then this is the book for you.

This is not yet another get-fit-quick program. It's a look at the things which have prevented you in the past from becoming the fit, active person you've always wanted to be, and a source of advice, inspiration and ideas to help you overcome those things this time around. Change your habits and attitude to exercise for good.

Too tired? Lacking motivation? Bored by exercise? You won't be after reading this book!

"Joanne is a true inspiration! Her passion, commitment and no nonsense attitude never fails to motivate her clients to get moving and achieve their health and fitness goals"

Sarah Price, triathlete and five times Ironman finisher

Paperback – ISBN 978-0-9933388-0-9
e-book – ISBN 978-0-9933388-1-6

Also in this series

What's Your Excuse for not Living a Life You Love?

Monica Castenetto
Overcome your excuses and lead a happier, more fulfilling life

Are you stuck in a life you don't love? Have you reached a point where your life doesn't feel right for you any-more? Then this book is for you.

This is not yet another self-help book claiming to re-veal the secret to permanent happiness. Instead, it helps you to tackle the things which have been holding you back and gives ideas, advice and inspiration to help you move on to a better life.

Don't know what you want? Scared of failure? Hate change? Worried about what others might think? This book will help you overcome all of your excuses and give you the motivation you need to change your life.

"Monica's energy, enthusiasm for life and her

*grounded, supportive coaching style never fail to
stimulate and inspire her clients to find ways to live a
life they love"*

Nicci Bonfanti, Master Trainer and Coach

Paperback – ISBN 978-0-9933388-4-7
e-book – ISBN 978-0-9933388-5-4